# Carb Cycling Diet Plan and Cookbook

*Delicious Recipes for Weight Loss, Muscle Building and Maintaining Energy Levels*

**JOY JIM**

# Table of Contents

# INTRODUCTION

Carbohydrates, a dietary mainstay for many, have sparked considerable controversy in recent times. While some advocate for their necessity in fueling the body and promoting overall health, others tout the merits of low-carb diets for weight management and vitality. Yet, there exists a third path that merges the advantages of both high- and low-carb approaches: **carb cycling**.

Carb cycling stands as a dietary tactic involving the rotation between days of high, low, and moderate carbohydrate intake, aiming to optimize metabolism, facilitate weight loss, and enhance physical performance. Through the manipulation of carbohydrate consumption, carb cycling facilitates the utilization of stored fat for energy while safeguarding muscle mass and fostering holistic wellness.

At the core of carb cycling lays the premise that the body responds differently to varying carbohydrate levels. During high-carb days, carbohydrates serve as the primary fuel source, fostering glycogen storage in muscles and the liver. This proves particularly advantageous for athletes and those partaking in rigorous physical endeavors, given that glycogen stands as a readily accessible energy reservoir.

Conversely, low-carb days prompt the body to rely on alternative fuel sources like stored fat and ketones. This metabolic shift, termed **ketosis,** has demonstrated efficacy in promoting weight loss, enhancing insulin sensitivity, and mitigating inflammation. By alternating between high and low-carb days, carb cycling enables individuals to harness the benefits of both approaches, establishing a harmonious and sustainable dietary regimen.

Carb cycling emerges as a versatile dietary strategy adaptable to diverse individuals, including:

**Weight Management Aspirants:** Carb cycling facilitates weight loss by fostering fat reduction while preserving muscle mass. Moreover, high-carb days offer the opportunity to indulge in favorite carbohydrate-rich foods in moderation, diminishing feelings of deprivation and bolstering adherence to the diet.

**Athletes and Fitness Enthusiasts:** Carb cycling can amplify athletic performance by ensuring ample glycogen reserves for high-intensity activities. Additionally, it supports recovery by curbing inflammation and aiding muscle repair.

**Individuals with Insulin Resistance:** Carb cycling holds promise in enhancing insulin sensitivity, rendering it a viable approach for managing conditions like type-2 diabetes and metabolic syndrome.

**Advocates of a Balanced Lifestyle:** Carb cycling presents a flexible and sustainable dietary regimen customizable to individual needs and preferences. Its inclusivity of a diverse array of foods fosters long-term adherence and overall well-being.

In essence, carb cycling emerges as a potent dietary methodology amalgamating the strengths of high- and low-carb diets, furnishing a balanced and sustainable blueprint for weight management, athletic prowess, and holistic health. By grasping the fundamentals of carb cycling and tailoring the approach to your requirements, you can unlock its full transformative potential.

Subsequent chapters will delve deeper into the science behind carb cycling, explore assorted protocols, and furnish comprehensive meal plans and recipes to facilitate your initiation into the world of carb cycling.

Whether you're a novice or a seasoned dieter, this guide is crafted to equip you with the insights and resources essential for making carb cycling a triumph in your life.

# PART: 1 THE SCIENTIFIC FOUNDATION OF CARB CYCLING

## Understanding Macronutrients

Carb cycling, is designed to optimize metabolic function, facilitate weight loss, and bolster athletic performance. To execute carb cycling effectively, it's imperative to comprehend the fundamental principles of macronutrients and their impacts on the body.

Macronutrients, commonly referred to as macros, encompass carbohydrates, fats, and proteins, serving as primary sources of energy and supporting various physiological processes. These nutrients are consumed in substantial quantities and are indispensable for overall health and vitality. In contrast, micronutrients, such as vitamins and minerals, are ingested in smaller proportions and predominantly facilitate biochemical reactions within the body.

Carbohydrates, serving as the body's primary energy reservoir, play a pivotal role in promoting optimal health and maximizing fitness levels. Upon consumption of carb-rich foods, they undergo breakdown into simple sugar molecules, notably glucose, which enters the bloodstream and subsequently undergoes conversion into energy in the form of ATP. Surplus glucose not immediately utilized for energy may be stored as glycogen in the muscles and liver, earmarked for future utilization, particularly during periods of intense physical exertion.

Proteins are indispensable for the repair and maintenance of all bodily tissues, encompassing muscles, bones, skin, and other vital structures. Additionally, they facilitate the production of essential hormones and enzymes crucial for supporting the immune system. When mobilized as an energy source, proteins are typically metabolized once carbohydrate and fat reserves in the body have been depleted.

Fats, often subject to misconceptions, are imperative for optimal bodily functioning. Healthy fats aid in the absorption of vitamins, furnish the body with essential fatty acids it cannot synthesize, and contribute to the flavor and texture of foods. Nonetheless, not all fats are created equal, and it's advisable to substitute saturated and trans fats with healthier unsaturated fats sourced from plants, such as nuts, avocados, and olive oil.

In the realm of carb cycling, comprehending the significance of macronutrients is paramount for crafting a meal plan aligned with your objectives. On high-carb days, prioritize whole-grain carbohydrates like oatmeal, brown rice, quinoa, and sweet potatoes, complemented by lean meats, eggs, or plant-based protein sources. Conversely, on low-carb days opt for low-glycemic carbohydrates such as leafy green vegetables, legumes, nuts, and seeds, alongside lean meats or plant-based proteins.

It's imperative to seek guidance from a healthcare professional before embarking on any new dietary regimen to ascertain its safety and suitability for your individual requirements.

## The Roles of Carbohydrates in Body

Carbohydrates play a pivotal role in the body as the primary source of energy for various physiological processes. Upon consumption, carbohydrates undergo breakdown into glucose, which enters the bloodstream and is utilized either for immediate energy, stored as glycogen for future use, or stored as fat. This glucose is indispensable for fueling both bodily activities and cognitive functions, ensuring optimal performance and cognitive acuity.

Complex carbohydrates, such as those found in cereals, legumes, and potatoes, offer sustained energy due to their prolonged digestion process compared to simple carbohydrates. Incorporating nutrient-rich carbohydrate sources like vegetables and fruits into one's diet provides essential vitamins, minerals, and fiber, which contribute to overall health and well-being.

### Insight into Insulin Mechanisms

Insulin, a hormone synthesized by the pancreas, plays a pivotal role in regulating blood sugar levels and facilitating the uptake of glucose into cells for energy production or storage. Elevated carbohydrate intake prompts increased insulin secretion to manage heightened glucose levels. However, excessive insulin production stemming from a carbohydrate-rich diet can precipitate weight gain, insulin resistance, and elevate the risk of conditions like type 2 diabetes and heart disease.

### *Strategic Management through Carb Cycling*

Carb cycling offers a systematic approach to regulating insulin levels by alternating between high-carb and low-carb days. By cycling carbohydrates, individuals afford their bodies the opportunity to utilize fat as an energy source alongside glucose, potentially enhancing insulin sensitivity and mitigating the risk of insulin-related health complications.

### *Benefits of Carb Cycling*

Carb cycling presents myriad benefits for individuals striving to optimize their weight, fitness objectives, and overall health. By oscillating between low and high carb days, carb cycling aids in weight management, boosts athletic performance, and may enhance insulin sensitivity. Research indicates that carb cycling could be particularly advantageous for individuals grappling with insulin resistance, prediabetes, or encountering weight loss plateaus.

Furthermore, carb cycling enables individuals to maintain a balanced macronutrient intake while strategically adjusting carbohydrate consumption in accordance with activity levels and goals. By integrating carb cycling into their dietary regimen, individuals may potentially augment metabolic flexibility, elevate energy levels, and bolster overall well-being.

Appreciating the role of carbohydrates in bodily functions, comprehending the intricacies of insulin's impact on metabolism, and recognizing the advantages of carb cycling are pivotal for devising an effective and sustainable dietary plan aligned with individual health and fitness aspirations.

Leveraging the science behind carb cycling empowers individuals to optimize their nutritional intake, enhance performance, and attain enduring success in their wellness journey.

# PART 2: CARB CYCLING PROTOCOLS

Carb cycling, is tailored to support diverse health and fitness objectives. This approach is renowned for its efficacy in aiding weight loss, enhancing athletic performance, and ameliorating symptoms associated with chronic conditions like type-2 diabetes.

Carbohydrates are categorized into two types: simple and complex. Simple carbs comprise one or two sugar molecules, whereas complex carbs encompass three or more. Notable examples of complex carbs include starches found in cereals, legumes, and potatoes.

The flexibility of carb cycling lies in its adaptability to individual preferences and requirements, allowing for adjustments in carbohydrate consumption over alternating time frames. For instance, individuals may opt for high-carb, low-fat diets on specific days and vice versa.

At the core of carb cycling's efficacy lies its capacity to modulate insulin levels and glycogen reserves, potentially fostering improved insulin sensitivity and overall well-being. A 2013 study underscores the potential benefits of intermittent energy and carbohydrate restriction in enhancing insulin sensitivity and facilitating weight management.

While carb cycling holds promise for weight loss, performance enhancement, and chronic condition management, it is imperative to seek guidance from healthcare professionals before embarking on a new dietary regimen to assess potential health risks.

Embarking on a carb cycling journey necessitates determining daily caloric needs and macronutrient proportions tailored to your objectives and activity levels. Higher-carb days typically entail 40 to 50% carbohydrate intake and 25 to 35% protein, with lower-carb days reversing these ratios.

Crafting meals aligned with these macronutrient ratios is paramount for adhering to the carb cycling protocol. Higher-carb days emphasize whole-grain carbohydrates like oatmeal, brown rice, quinoa, and sweet potatoes, complemented by lean meats, eggs, or plant-based proteins. Conversely, lower-carb days prioritize low-glycemic carbohydrates such as leafy green vegetables, beans, legumes, nuts, and seeds, alongside lean meats or plant-based proteins.

Planning meals meticulously and predominantly cooking at home aids in meeting macronutrient targets, ensuring adherence to the rigors of carb cycling. The structured nature of this dietary approach underscores the importance of alternating between high and low-carb days to maximize its benefits.

In essence, carb cycling emerges as a versatile and adaptable dietary strategy conducive to achieving diverse health and fitness goals through strategic manipulation of carbohydrate intake. By comprehending the underlying science and adhering to prescribed guidelines, you can harness the potential of carb cycling to bolster your overall health and well-being.

## The Basics of Carb Cycling

Carb cycling is a dietary strategy that capitalizes on the understanding that the body responds differently to varying levels of carbohydrate intake.

During high-carb days, the body predominantly relies on carbohydrates as its primary energy source, fostering glycogen storage in muscles and the liver. This proves advantageous, particularly for athletes and those engaging in rigorous physical activity, as glycogen serves as readily available fuel.

Conversely, low-carb days prompt the body to resort to alternative energy sources like stored fat and ketones, inducing a metabolic state known as ketosis. Ketosis has been associated with benefits such as weight loss, improved insulin sensitivity, and reduced inflammation.

By oscillating between high-carb and low-carb days, carb cycling amalgamates the advantages of both approaches, culminating in a balanced and sustainable dietary regimen. The specifics of macronutrient ratios and calorie intake can vary based on individual goals, activity levels, and preferences.

A typical carb cycling protocol may involve high-carb days characterized by carbohydrate intake of 2-2.5 grams per pound of body weight, alongside moderate protein and lower fat intake. Conversely, low-carb days may feature carbohydrate intake of 0.5 grams per pound of body weight, with higher protein and fat consumption. Optionally, individuals may incorporate no-carb days with carbohydrate intake below 30 grams, accompanied by the highest protein and fat intake.

The frequency and duration of high-carb and low-carb days can be tailored to individual needs and preferences, with options ranging from weekly to daily or monthly cycles. It's imperative to recognize that carb cycling is not a one-size-fits-all approach. Please seek guidance from healthcare professionals or registered dietitians to devise personalized plans aligned with your specific goals and health status.

# Different Carb Cycling Protocols

Carb cycling offers various protocols tailored to individual goals and preferences, each involving alternating between high-carb and low-carb days. Understanding and selecting the right protocol is essential for optimizing results and adherence to the regimen.

**Weekly Carb Cycling**:

5 low-carb days followed by 2 high-carb days

4 low-carb days followed by 3 high-carb days

**Daily Carb Cycling:**

Alternating between high-carb and low-carb days, possibly including no-carb days

**Monthly Carb Cycling**:

2-3 weeks of low-carb days followed by 1 week of high-carb days

**Targeted Carb Cycling**:

Adjusting carb intake based on workout days vs. rest days, with higher carbs on workout days and lower carbs on rest days

The specific macronutrient ratios and calorie intake can vary based on individual goals, activity levels, and personal preferences. Experimentation may be necessary to find the protocol that suits you best.

## How to Choose the Right Protocol for You

**Goals:** Determine if you're aiming for weight loss, muscle gain, or improved athletic performance to align with a suitable protocol.

**Lifestyle and Activity Levels**: Choose a protocol that matches your activity levels, with more high-carb days for highly active individuals and fewer for sedentary individuals.

**Personal Preferences:** Select a protocol that fits your lifestyle, whether it's daily, weekly, or monthly cycling.

**Health Conditions**: Individuals with specific health conditions like diabetes may need to adjust their protocol to manage blood sugar levels effectively.

Consulting with a healthcare professional or registered dietitian can provide personalized guidance to choose the most appropriate carb cycling protocol.

As you progress, monitor your body's response and be prepared to adjust your plan accordingly. This may involve tweaking macronutrient ratios, changing the frequency of high-carb and low-carb days, or adjusting calorie intake based on your body's feedback.

Remember, successful carb cycling requires patience, consistency, and a willingness to adapt. By carefully tracking progress and making necessary adjustments, you can optimize your carb cycling plan to achieve your desired outcomes.

## Adjusting Your Carb Cycling Plan

As you embark on your carb cycling journey, remain attentive to your progress and be open to adjusting your plan as necessary. This may involve:

Fine-tuning macronutrient ratios on high-carb and low-carb days

Modifying the frequency of high-carb and low-carb days

Incorporating more or fewer no-carb days

Adapting calorie intake based on your body's response

By maintaining a close eye on your progress, listening to your body's cues, and making gradual adjustments, you can tailor your carb cycling plan to yield optimal outcomes.

# PART 3: MEAL PLANS FOR VARIOUS GOALS

These plans are carefully crafted to accommodate various carb cycling protocols and macronutrient ratios to effectively support your desired outcomes.

**Weight Loss Meal Plan**

For those on a weight loss journey, a carb cycling meal plan can be remarkably effective. Alternating between low-carb and high-carb days prompts the body to adapt to different energy sources, potentially leading to increased fat loss and enhanced insulin sensitivity.

Low-carb days: Concentrate on protein-rich foods, healthy fats, and low-carb vegetables like leafy greens and broccoli. Aim for 0.5-1 gram of carbs per pound of body weight.

High-carb days: Integrate complex carbohydrates such as whole grains, legumes, and fruits. Aim for 2-3 grams of carbs per pound of body weight.

**Muscle Gain Meal Plan**

Individuals aspiring to build muscle mass can benefit from a carb cycling meal plan, optimizing muscle growth and recovery. By consuming more carbohydrates on high-carb days, the body replenishes glycogen stores and supports muscle development.

Low-carb days: Emphasize protein-rich foods, healthy fats, and low-carb vegetables like leafy greens and broccoli. Aim for 0.5-1 gram of carbs per pound of body weight. High-carb days: Include complex carbohydrates such as whole grains, legumes, and fruits. Aim for 3-4 grams of carbs per pound of body weight.

**Maintenance Meal Plan**

For those aiming to maintain their current weight and body composition, a carb cycling meal plan fosters consistent energy levels and overall health. Alternating between low-carb and high-carb days helps the body adapt to diverse energy sources, promoting metabolic flexibility.

Low-carb days: Prioritize protein-rich foods, healthy fats, and low-carb vegetables like leafy greens and broccoli. Aim for 0.5-1 gram of carbs per pound of body weight. High-carb days: Include complex carbohydrates such as whole grains, legumes, and fruits. Aim for 2-3 grams of carbs per pound of body weight.

These meal plans serve as a foundational framework for individuals striving to achieve specific objectives. However, it's crucial to collaborate with a healthcare professional or registered dietitian to devise a personalized meal plan aligned with individual needs and preferences. Your unique journey deserves tailored guidance to ensure success.

Here's a breakdown of tailored meal plans for each goal, along with some helpful tips to guide you along the way:

## Weight Loss Meal Plan

When aiming to shed some pounds, having a well-structured meal plan is key. Here's how you can create one:

**Calorie Intake:** Trim your daily calorie intake by 500-1000 calories to initiate weight loss. This can involve portion control, avoiding calorie-dense foods, and increasing physical activity.

**Macronutrient Ratio:** Strive for a balanced diet with a ratio of 15-20% protein, 25-30% fat, and 55-60% carbohydrates, tailored to your preferences and needs.

**Food Choices:** Prioritize whole, unprocessed foods like fruits, veggies, lean proteins, and whole grains while steering clear of sugary drinks and processed foods.

**Meal Frequency:** Aim for 3-5 main meals and 2-3 snacks spread throughout the day to maintain energy levels and curb hunger.

**Hydration:** Hydrate yourself adequately with 8-10 glasses of water daily to support satiety and overall health.

## Muscle Gain Meal Plan

Consider the following:

**Calorie Intake:** Boost your daily calorie intake by 250-500 calories to fuel muscle growth, achieved through increased meal frequency and portion sizes.

**Macronutrient Ratio:** Aim for a ratio of 20-25% protein, 30-35% fat, and 45-50% carbohydrates, catering to your individual requirements.

**Food Choices:** Opt for lean proteins like chicken and fish, complex carbs such as brown rice and sweet potatoes, and incorporate healthy fats for added nourishment.

**Meal Frequency:** Aim for 5-7 main meals and 2-3 snacks throughout the day to support muscle recovery and sustain energy levels.

**Hydration:** Stay hydrated with 8-10 glasses of water daily to aid muscle recovery and overall well-being.

## Maintenance Meal Plan

For maintaining your current weight and physique, sustaining a balanced meal plan is vital. Here's how you can achieve that:

**Calorie Intake:** Maintain a consistent calorie intake to support overall health and well-being.

**Macronutrient Ratio:** Aim for a balanced diet with a ratio of 15-20% protein, 25-30% fat, and 55-60% carbohydrates, adjusted based on your preferences.

**Food Choices:** Stick to whole, unprocessed foods and avoid sugary drinks and refined carbohydrates.

**Meal Frequency:** Aim for 3-5 main meals and 2-3 snacks evenly spaced throughout the day to prevent excessive hunger and maintain energy levels.

**Hydration:** Hydrate adequately with 8-10 glasses of water daily to support overall health.

## Meal Planning Tips and Tricks

Regardless of your specific goal, here are some universal tips to streamline your meal planning process:

**Plan Ahead:** Create a weekly meal plan and grocery list in advance to ensure healthy choices and avoid impulsive decisions.

**KISS: Keep It Simple, Silly! :** Opt for simple, time-efficient meals that can be prepared in less than 30 minutes.

**Incorporate Healthy Fats:** Include sources of healthy fats like avocado and nuts to enhance satiety and overall health.

**Eat Mindfully:** Listen to your body's hunger and fullness cues, eat slowly, and savor each bite to foster a healthier relationship with food.

**Seek Support:** Share your meal plans with loved ones for encouragement and accountability.

**Flexibility:** Allow room for flexibility in your meal plan and make adjustments as needed based on individual preferences and circumstances.

**Track Progress:** Keep track of your meals and progress using a food diary or meal tracking app to stay on course.

**Consultation:** Consider consulting with a registered dietitian or healthcare professional to tailor a personalized meal plan that aligns with your goals and preferences.

# PART 4: DELICIOUS RECIPES



## Breakfast Recipes

Breakfast is like the morning's gentle nudge, setting the tone for the day ahead. Here, we've whipped up a collection of delicious and nutritious breakfast recipes to suit various tastes and dietary preferences:

## Low-Carb: Spinach and Feta Scrambled Eggs Serves: 1

Ingredients:

2 large eggs

1/4 cup fresh spinach leaves, chopped

1/4 cup crumbled feta cheese

Salt and pepper to taste

1 tablespoon olive oil

Instructions:

Crack the eggs into a bowl and whisk them with a fork, adding salt and pepper.

Heat olive oil in a non-stick pan over medium heat.

Pour the egg mixture into the pan and scramble until nearly set.

Add chopped spinach and crumbled feta cheese to the pan, stirring to combine.

Cook for another minute until the eggs are fully set and the spinach is wilted.

Serve hot and enjoy!

Nutrition Information (per serving): Calories: 240 Protein: 18g Fat: 18g Carbohydrates: 4g Fiber: 2g Sugar: 1g Sodium: 250mg

## Low-Carb: Coconut Flour Pancakes Serves: 1

Ingredients:

1/2 cup coconut flour

1/4 cup almond flour

1/4 cup granulated sweetener (such as Swerve or Erythritol)

2 large eggs

1/2 cup unsweetened almond milk

1/4 teaspoon salt

1/4 teaspoon baking soda

1 tablespoon melted coconut oil

1 teaspoon vanilla extract

Instructions:

Combine coconut flour, almond flour, sweetener, and salt in a bowl.

In another bowl, whisk eggs, almond milk, and melted coconut oil.

Mix wet ingredients into dry until a batter forms.

Heat a non-stick pan over medium heat and drop batter by 1/4 cupful.

Cook for 2-3 minutes until bubbles form, then flip and cook for another 1-2 minutes.

Serve hot with desired toppings.

Nutrition Information (per serving): Calories: 320 Protein: 6g Fat: 26g Carbohydrates: 6g Fiber: 4g Sugar: 1g Sodium: 200mg

# Moderate Carb: Avocado Toast with Poached Eggs Serves: 1

Ingredients:

1 slice whole-grain bread

1/2 avocado, mashed

2 poached eggs

Salt and pepper to taste

Optional: red pepper flakes, chopped fresh herbs

**Instructions:**

Toast the bread until lightly browned.

Spread mashed avocado on top.

Poach eggs until whites are set and yolks reach desired doneness.

Place poached eggs on avocado toast and season with salt, pepper, and optional toppings.

Serve hot and enjoy!

**Nutrition Information (per serving)**: Calories: 350 Protein: 14g Fat: 24g Carbohydrates: 20g Fiber: 7g Sugar: 2g Sodium: 200mg

## Moderate Carb: Greek Yogurt Parfait with Granola Serves: 1

Ingredients:

1 cup Greek yogurt

1/4 cup granola

1/2 cup mixed berries

1 tablespoon honey or maple syrup (optional)

Instructions:

Layer Greek yogurt, granola, and mixed berries in a bowl.

Drizzle with honey or maple syrup if desired.

Serve chilled and enjoy!

Nutrition Information (per serving): Calories: 250 Protein: 20g Fat: 10g Carbohydrates: 30g Fiber: 4g Sugar: 20g Sodium: 50mg

## High Carb: Overnight Oats with Banana and Almond Butter Serves: 1

Ingredients:

1/2 cup rolled oats

1/2 cup unsweetened almond milk

1/2 banana, sliced

2 tablespoons almond butter

1 tablespoon honey or maple syrup (optional)

Pinch of salt

Instructions:

Combine oats, almond milk, banana, and almond butter in a jar.

Stir well and refrigerate overnight or for at least 4 hours.

In the morning, add honey or maple syrup if desired.

Serve chilled and enjoy!

Nutrition Information (per serving): Calories: 400 Protein: 8g Fat: 20g Carbohydrates: 60g Fiber: 8g Sugar: 30g Sodium: 50mg

# Lunch Recipes

## Low Carb: Chicken Caesar Salad Servings:1

Ingredients:

1 pound cooked chicken breast, diced

2 cups romaine lettuce, chopped

1/4 cup Caesar dressing (homemade or store-bought)

1/4 cup croutons (homemade or store-bought)

1/4 cup shaved Parmesan cheese

Salt and pepper to taste

Instructions:

In a large bowl, combine the chopped romaine lettuce, diced chicken breast, and croutons.

Drizzle the Caesar dressing over the top and toss to combine.

Sprinkle the shaved Parmesan cheese over the top and season with salt and pepper to taste.

Serve immediately and enjoy!

Nutrition Information (per serving): Calories: 320 Protein: 35g Fat: 20g Carbohydrates: 5g Fiber: 2g Sugar: 2g Sodium: 400mg

## Low Carb: Tuna Salad Lettuce Wraps
## Servings: 1

Ingredients:

1 can of tuna (drained and flaked)

1/4 cup mayonnaise

1/4 cup chopped onion

1/4 cup chopped celery

1/4 cup chopped hard-boiled egg

2 cups lettuce leaves

Salt and pepper to taste

Instructions:

In a medium bowl, combine the tuna, mayonnaise, chopped onion, chopped celery, and chopped hard-boiled egg.

Mix well until all the ingredients are fully incorporated.

Spoon the tuna salad onto the lettuce leaves and season with salt and pepper to taste.

Serve immediately and enjoy!

Nutrition Information (per serving): Calories: 250 Protein: 30g Fat: 15g Carbohydrates: 5g Fiber: 2g Sugar: 2g Sodium: 300mg

# Moderate Carb: Quinoa Salad with Grilled Chicken Servings: 1

Ingredients:

1 cup cooked quinoa

1 pound grilled chicken breast, diced

1 cup mixed vegetables (such as cherry tomatoes, cucumber, and bell peppers)

2 tablespoons olive oil

1 tablespoon lemon juice

Salt and pepper to taste

Instructions:

In a large bowl, combine the cooked quinoa, diced grilled chicken, and mixed vegetables.

Drizzle the olive oil and lemon juice over the top and toss to combine.

Season with salt and pepper to taste.

Serve immediately and enjoy!

Nutrition Information (per serving): Calories: 400 Protein: 35g Fat: 20g Carbohydrates: 40g Fiber: 5g Sugar: 5g Sodium: 400mg

## Moderate Carb: Turkey and Avocado Sandwich on Whole Grain Servings: 1

Ingredients:

2 slices whole grain bread

2 ounces sliced turkey breast

1/2 avocado, sliced

1 cup mixed greens

1/4 cup sliced red onion

1/4 cup sliced cucumber

1 tablespoon mayonnaise

Salt and pepper to taste

Instructions:

Lay the slices of whole grain bread on a flat surface.

Spread the mayonnaise on one slice of bread.

Top with the sliced turkey breast, sliced avocado, mixed greens, sliced red onion, and sliced cucumber.

Top with the second slice of bread.

Serve immediately and enjoy!

Nutrition Information (per serving): Calories: 500 Protein: 35g Fat: 25g Carbohydrates: 40g Fiber: 10g Sugar: 5g Sodium: 400mg

## High Carb: Whole Wheat Pasta with Roasted Vegetables and Pesto Servings: 1

Ingredients:

1 cup cooked whole wheat pasta

1 cup roasted vegetables (such as zucchini, bell peppers, and cherry tomatoes)

1/4 cup pesto sauce

1/4 cup grated Parmesan cheese

Salt and pepper to taste

Instructions:

Cook the whole wheat pasta according to the package instructions.

Toss the cooked pasta with the roasted vegetables and pesto sauce.

Sprinkle the grated Parmesan cheese over the top and season with salt and pepper to taste.

Serve immediately and enjoy!

Nutrition Information (per serving): Calories: 600 Protein: 15g Fat: 20g Carbohydrates: 80g Fiber: 10g Sugar: 10g Sodium: 400mg

# Dinner Recipes

## Low Carb: Chicken Caesar Salad Servings: 1

Ingredients:

1 pound cooked chicken breast, diced

2 cups romaine lettuce, chopped

1/4 cup Caesar dressing (homemade or store-bought)

1/4 cup croutons (homemade or store-bought)

1/4 cup shaved Parmesan cheese

Salt and pepper to taste

Instructions:

In a large bowl, combine the chopped romaine lettuce, diced chicken breast, and croutons.

Drizzle the Caesar dressing over the top and toss to combine.

Sprinkle the shaved Parmesan cheese over the top and season with salt and pepper to taste.

Serve immediately and enjoy!

Nutrition Information (per serving): Calories: 320 Protein: 35g Fat: 20g Carbohydrates: 5g Fiber: 2g Sugar: 2g Sodium: 400mg

# Low Carb: Tuna Salad Lettuce Wraps

Servings: 1

Ingredients:

1 can of tuna (drained and flaked)

1/4 cup mayonnaise

1/4 cup chopped onion

1/4 cup chopped celery

1/4 cup chopped hard-boiled egg

2 cups lettuce leaves

Salt and pepper to taste

Instructions:

In a medium bowl, combine the tuna, mayonnaise, chopped onion, chopped celery, and chopped hard-boiled egg.

Mix well until all the ingredients are fully incorporated.

Spoon the tuna salad onto the lettuce leaves and season with salt and pepper to taste.

Serve immediately and enjoy!

Nutrition Information (per serving): Calories: 250 Protein: 30g Fat: 15g Carbohydrates: 5g Fiber: 2g Sugar: 2g Sodium: 300mg

# Moderate Carb: Quinoa Salad with Grilled Chicken Servings: 1

Ingredients:

1 cup cooked quinoa

1 pound grilled chicken breast, diced

1 cup mixed vegetables (such as cherry tomatoes, cucumber, and bell peppers)

2 tablespoons olive oil

1 tablespoon lemon juice

Salt and pepper to taste

Instructions:

In a large bowl, combine the cooked quinoa, diced grilled chicken, and mixed vegetables.

Drizzle the olive oil and lemon juice over the top and toss to combine.

Season with salt and pepper to taste.

Serve immediately and enjoy!

Nutrition Information (per serving): Calories: 400 Protein: 35g Fat: 20g Carbohydrates: 40g Fiber: 5g Sugar: 5g Sodium: 400mg

## Moderate Carb: Baked Salmon with Sweet Potatoes and Broccoli Servings: 1

Ingredients:

1 pound salmon fillet

1 large sweet potato, peeled and cubed

1 cup broccoli florets

2 tablespoons olive oil

Salt and pepper to taste

Instructions:

Preheat the oven to 400°F (200°C).

Line a baking sheet with parchment paper.

Place the sweet potato cubes on the baking sheet and drizzle with olive oil.

Roast the sweet potatoes in the oven for 20-25 minutes, or until they are tender and lightly browned.

Place the salmon fillet on the baking sheet and drizzle with olive oil.

Roast the salmon in the oven for 12-15 minutes, or until it is cooked through.

Toss the broccoli florets with olive oil, salt, and pepper.

Roast the broccoli in the oven for 5-7 minutes, or until it is tender and lightly browned.

Serve the salmon with the roasted sweet potatoes and broccoli.

Nutrition Information (per serving): Calories: 400 Protein: 35g Fat: 20g Carbohydrates: 30g Fiber: 5g Sugar: 5g Sodium: 400mg

## Moderate Carb: Chicken and Quinoa Bowl with Roasted Vegetables Servings: 1

Ingredients:

1 pound cooked chicken breast, diced

1 cup cooked quinoa

1 cup roasted vegetables (such as Brussels sprouts, asparagus, and red bell peppers)

2 tablespoons olive oil

Salt and pepper to taste

Instructions:

Cook the quinoa according to the package instructions.

Toss the roasted vegetables with olive oil, salt, and pepper.

Serve the cooked chicken breast on top of the quinoa and roasted vegetables.

Nutrition Information (per serving): Calories: 400 Protein: 35g Fat: 20g Carbohydrates: 30g Fiber: 5g Sugar: 5g Sodium: 400mg

## Low Carb: Celery with Almond Butter and Raisins.

Serving: 1

Ingredients:

2 stalks celery

2 tablespoons almond butter

1/4 cup raisins

Salt to taste

Instructions:

Cut the celery into sticks.

Spread 1 tablespoon of almond butter on each celery stick.

Top with 1/4 cup of raisins.

Serve immediately and enjoy!

Nutrition Information (per serving):

Calories: 150

Protein: 4g

Fat: 12g

Carbohydrates: 10g

Fiber: 2g

Sugar: 6g

Sodium: 50mg

## Low Carb: Cucumber Slices with Hummus

Servings: 1

Ingredients:

1 cucumber

2 tablespoons hummus

Salt to taste

Instructions:

Cut the cucumber into slices.

Spread 1 tablespoon of hummus on each cucumber slice.

Serve immediately and enjoy!

Nutrition Information (per serving):

Calories: 100

Protein: 2g

Fat: 10g

Carbohydrates: 6g

Fiber: 2g

Sugar: 2g

Sodium: 50mg

## Moderate Carb: Apple Slices with Peanut Butter

Servings: 1

Ingredients:

1 apple

2 tablespoons peanut butter

Salt to taste

Instructions:

Cut the apple into slices.

Spread 1 tablespoon of peanut butter on each apple slice.

Serve immediately and enjoy!

Nutrition Information (per serving):

Calories: 200

Protein: 8g

Fat: 16g

Carbohydrates: 20g

Fiber: 4g

Sugar: 12g

Sodium: 50mg

## Moderate Carb: Greek Yogurt with Berries and Honey

Servings: 1

Ingredients:

1 cup Greek yogurt

1/2 cup mixed berries

1 tablespoon honey

Salt to taste

Instructions:

Mix the Greek yogurt, mixed berries, and honey together in a bowl.

Serve immediately and enjoy!

Nutrition Information (per serving):

Calories: 200

Protein: 20g

Fat: 0g

Carbohydrates: 40g

Fiber: 4g

Sugar: 20g

Sodium: 50mg

## High Carb: Rice Cakes with Avocado and Tomato

Servings: 1

Ingredients:

2 rice cakes

1/2 avocado, mashed

1 tomato, sliced

Salt to taste

Instructions:

Toast the rice cakes.

Spread 1/2 avocado on each rice cake.

Top with 1 tomato slice.

Serve immediately and enjoy!

Nutrition Information (per serving):

Calories: 400

Protein: 4g

Fat: 20g

Carbohydrates: 60g

Fiber: 10g

Sugar: 10g

Sodium: 50mg

# PART 5: CARB CYCLING FOR SPECIAL DIETARY NEEDS

Carb cycling can also be adapted to accommodate special dietary needs, including vegetarianism.

Carb Cycling for Vegetarians

Carb cycling, isn't just for omnivores. It can be effectively adopted by vegetarians and vegans to optimize metabolism, aid weight loss, and enhance athletic performance. Here's how vegetarians can make the most of carb cycling:

Challenges for Vegetarians: A primary challenge for vegetarians lies in sourcing sufficient protein. Unlike omnivores who have access to animal-based protein sources, vegetarians rely on plant-based options, which may have lower protein content. Balancing macronutrient ratios can also be tricky.

Strategies for Vegetarians:

**High-Protein Plant-Based Foods:** Incorporate legumes, lentils, tofu, and tempeh into meals for adequate protein.

**Combine Protein Sources:** Mix different plant-based proteins, like legumes and whole grains, for a well-rounded amino acid profile.

**Incorporate Healthy Fats:** Avocado, nuts, and seeds not only offer healthy fats but also provide energy.

**Monitor Macronutrient Ratios:** Keep an eye on the balance of protein, carbs, and fats in each meal to meet nutritional needs.

**Consult a Registered Dietitian:** Seek guidance from a registered dietitian to tailor a carb cycling plan to individual dietary requirements.

Sample Meal Plan for Vegetarians:

**Low-Carb Day:**

Breakfast: Oatmeal with almond milk, banana, and walnuts

Lunch: Lentil soup with whole-grain bread and a side salad

Dinner: Grilled tofu with roasted vegetables and quinoa

**High-Carb Day:**

Breakfast: Whole-grain waffles with mixed berries and yogurt

Lunch: Whole-grain pasta with marinara sauce and steamed broccoli

Dinner: Grilled portobello mushrooms with roasted sweet potatoes and green beans

By implementing these strategies and meal plans, vegetarians can effectively harness the benefits of carb cycling while maintaining their plant-based lifestyle.

# Carb Cycling for Vegans

Carb cycling for vegans involves adjusting carbohydrate intake based on energy needs while ensuring sufficient protein and fat intake from plant-based sources. Here are some tips for vegans when carb cycling:

**Focus on Whole Grains:** Whole grains like brown rice, quinoa, and whole wheat bread provide sustained energy and are rich in fiber and nutrients.

**Incorporate Legumes:** Lentils, chickpeas, and black beans are high in protein and fiber, making them excellent choices for vegans to meet their nutritional needs.

**Choose Plant-Based Protein Sources:** Tofu, tempeh, and seitan are all high in protein and can be used as alternatives to meat to ensure adequate protein intake.

**Monitor Carbohydrate Intake:** Aim to consume 2-3 grams of carbohydrates per pound of body weight per day, focusing on whole grains and legumes while being mindful of portion sizes.

**Incorporate Healthy Fats:** Avocados, nuts, and seeds are rich in healthy fats and can support overall health and well-being when included in the diet.

## Carb Cycling for Gluten-Free Diets

For individuals following gluten-free diets, carb cycling can still be effectively implemented. Here are some tips specific to carb cycling for gluten-free diets:

**Focus on Whole Grains:** Opt for naturally gluten-free whole grains like brown rice, quinoa, and corn to provide sustained energy and essential nutrients.

**Incorporate Legumes:** Legumes such as lentils, chickpeas, and black beans are naturally gluten-free and offer both protein and fiber for a balanced diet.

**Choose Gluten-Free Protein Sources:** Tofu, tempeh, and seitan are gluten-free protein options that can be included in meals to meet protein needs.

**Monitor Carbohydrate Intake:** Aim for 2-3 grams of carbohydrates per pound of body weight per day, prioritizing gluten-free whole grains and legumes.

**Include Healthy Fats:** Avocados, nuts, and seeds are excellent sources of healthy fats that can be incorporated into gluten-free meals to enhance flavor and provide essential nutrients.

# Carb Cycling for Dairy-Free Diets

For those following dairy-free diets, carb cycling can still be beneficial. Here are some tips for carb cycling on a dairy-free diet:

**Focus on Whole Grains:** Choose whole grains such as brown rice, quinoa, and whole wheat bread to provide complex carbohydrates and essential nutrients.

**Incorporate Legumes:** Legumes like lentils, chickpeas, and black beans are dairy-free protein sources that offer both protein and fiber for a balanced diet.

**Choose Dairy-Free Protein Sources:** Tofu, tempeh, and seitan are dairy-free protein options that can be used as substitutes for meat in meals.

**Monitor Carbohydrate Intake:** Aim for 2-3 grams of carbohydrates per pound of body weight per day, focusing on dairy-free whole grains and legumes.

**Include Healthy Fats:** Avocados, nuts, and seeds are dairy-free sources of healthy fats that can be included in meals to support overall health and well-being.

# PART 6: TIPS AND TRICKS FOR SUCCESS

## How to Stay on Track with Carb Cycling:

Plan Ahead: Prepare meals and snacks in advance to avoid impulsive decisions.

Track Your Progress: Use a food diary or tracking app to monitor carb intake and adjust as needed.

Stay Hydrated: Drinking water helps control hunger and supports overall health.

Get Enough Sleep: Aim for 7-9 hours per night to regulate hunger hormones.

Find Healthy Alternatives: Seek out substitutes for favorite foods to stay on track without feeling deprived.

Be Patient: Understand that results take time, and consistency is key.

How to Handle Social Situations:

Plan Ahead: Prepare for social events by knowing your options in advance.

Bring a Healthy Option: Take along a nutritious dish to ensure you have something suitable to eat.

Communicate with Others: Let friends and family know about your dietary needs to receive support.

Don't Be Afraid to Say No: Decline foods that don't align with your goals without feeling guilty.

Find Support: Seek encouragement from loved ones or professionals to help navigate social challenges.

How to Adjust Your Plan as Needed:

Listen to Your Body: Pay attention to how you feel and adjust your plan accordingly.

Monitor Your Progress: Regularly assess your results and be willing to make changes.

Be Flexible: Life is unpredictable, so adapt your plan as necessary.

Seek Professional Help: If struggling, consult with a healthcare provider or dietitian for guidance.

How to Track Your Progress:

Keep a Food Diary: Record meals and snacks to monitor carb intake.

Take Progress Videos: Visualize changes in your body over time.

Measure Your Progress: Track weight, body fat percentage, and other health metrics.

Celebrate Your Successes: Acknowledge achievements and learn from setbacks to stay motivated.

# CONCLUSION

Carb cycling emerges as a potent strategy for weight management and overall health enhancement. Through a thorough grasp of its underlying principles and dedicated application, you can unlock profound transformations in your well-being.

**The Power of Consistency:**

Consistency stands as the cornerstone of success in carb cycling. It is imperative to adhere steadfastly to the prescribed plan, making necessary adjustments along the journey to ensure alignment with nutritional needs. By maintaining consistency, you witness tangible results and solidify lasting changes in your health.

**The Future of Carb Cycling:**

The trajectory of carb cycling is promising, with ongoing research and advancements in nutrition and exercise science continually refining our understanding. As knowledge deepens regarding the nuanced interplay between diet, metabolism, and health, we anticipate the emergence of even more tailored and effective approaches to carb cycling.

**Final Thoughts and Next Steps:**

In summation, carb cycling offers a compelling avenue for weight loss and health optimization. By comprehending its principles and integrating them into your lifestyle with diligence, you can experience profound improvements in your overall well-being. Remember to prioritize consistency, exercise patience, and adapt the approach as necessary to meet evolving needs.

**Next Steps:**

**Initiate Consultation:** Seek guidance from a healthcare professional or registered dietitian to ascertain the suitability of carb cycling for your unique circumstances and to craft a personalized plan.

**Commence with Low-Carb Phase:** Begin your carb cycling journey with a phase focused on reduced carbohydrate intake, gradually adjusting as your body adapts.

**Monitor and Adjust:** Regularly assess progress and refine your plan to ensure it remains aligned with your evolving nutritional requirements and health goals.

**Embrace Consistency:** Maintain unwavering commitment to your carb cycling regimen, making necessary tweaks to sustain progress and achieve desired outcomes.

**Leverage Support Networks:** Seek encouragement and guidance from peers, family, or professionals to bolster your journey and navigate challenges effectively.

By adhering to these comprehensive steps and staying dedicated to your objectives, you pave the way for success with carb cycling, fostering a lifestyle characterized by improved health, vitality, and overall well-being.

# APPENDIX

## Carb Cycling Shopping List

Proteins:

Lean meats (chicken, turkey, fish)

Eggs

Tofu

Legumes (lentils, chickpeas, black beans)

Nuts and seeds (almonds, walnuts, chia seeds)

Vegetables:

Leafy greens (spinach, kale, collard greens)

Cruciferous vegetables (broccoli, cauliflower, Brussels sprouts)

Colorful vegetables (bell peppers, carrots, tomatoes)

Root vegetables (sweet potatoes, carrots, beets)

Fruits:

Berries (strawberries, blueberries, raspberries)

Citrus fruits (oranges, grapefruits, lemons)

Apples and pears

Avocados

Whole grains:

Brown rice

Quinoa

Whole wheat bread

Whole grain pasta

Healthy fats:

Avocado oil

Olive oil

Coconut oil

Nuts and seeds (almonds, walnuts, chia seeds)

Condiments:

Salt

Pepper

Herbs (basil, oregano, thyme)

Spices (cumin, coriander, turmeric)

**Carb Cycling Foods to Avoid:**

Refined carbohydrates:

White bread

Pasta

Rice

Cereals

Sugary foods:

Candy

Cookies

Cake

Ice cream

Processed meats:

Hot dogs

Sausages

Bacon

Ham

Fried foods:

French fries

Fried chicken

Fried fish

Fried vegetables

High-sugar drinks:

Soda

Sports drinks

Energy drinks

Fruit juices

## Carb Cycling Meal Prep Ideas:

Breakfast:

Overnight oats with fruit and nuts

Scrambled eggs with spinach and feta

Avocado toast with scrambled eggs

Lunch:

Grilled chicken breast with roasted vegetables

Quinoa salad with grilled chicken and vegetables

Lentil soup with whole grain bread

Dinner:

Grilled salmon with roasted asparagus and brown rice

Chicken stir-fry with vegetables and brown rice

Beef and vegetable kebabs with quinoa

## Carb Cycling Recipes for Kids:

Breakfast:

Peanut butter banana toast

Scrambled eggs with whole wheat toast

Yogurt parfait with granola and berries

Lunch:

Turkey and cheese wrap with carrot sticks

Chicken quesadilla with mixed greens

Grilled cheese sandwich with tomato soup

Dinner:

Chicken tenders with dipping sauce

Mac and cheese with a side of steamed broccoli

Grilled cheese and tomato sandwich with a side of carrot sticks

## Carb Cycling FAQs:

**Q: What is carb cycling?** A: Carb cycling is a diet that involves alternating between high-carb and low-carb days to help the body adapt to different energy sources.

**Q: How do I start carb cycling?** A: Start by consulting with a healthcare professional or registered dietitian to determine if carb cycling is right for you and to create a personalized plan.

**Q: What are some common mistakes to avoid when carb cycling?** A: Some common mistakes to avoid when carb cycling include not planning ahead, not tracking your progress, and not adjusting your plan as needed.

**Q: Can I still eat my favorite foods while carb cycling?** A: Yes, you can still eat your favorite foods while carb cycling, but you may need to make some adjustments to your portion sizes and frequency of consumption.

**Q: How long does it take to see results from carb cycling?** A: It can take several weeks to see results from carb cycling, as the body needs time to adapt to the new diet.

**Q: Can I do carb cycling with a busy schedule?** A: Yes, you can do carb cycling with a busy schedule by planning ahead, meal prepping, and making healthy choices when you're on-the-go.

# Glossary

A

Adaptation: Adjustments the body makes in response to changes in its environment.

Aerobic Exercise: Physical activity requiring oxygen, like running or swimming.

Alkaline: Having a pH level higher than 7.0, often associated with the alkaline diet.

Alkaline Diet: Emphasizes alkaline foods such as fruits, vegetables, and whole grains.

B

Beta-Hydroxy beta-Methylbutyrate (HMB): A leucine metabolite with anti-catabolic effects.

Blood Sugar: Glucose levels in the blood.

Body Fat Percentage: Percentage of body weight composed of fat.

Body Mass Index (BMI): Body fat measurement based on height and weight.


C

Carbohydrate: Macronutrient providing energy.

Carb Cycling: Alternating between high-carb and low-carb days.

Carb Load: Eating lots of carbs to replenish energy.

Catabolic: Muscle tissue breakdown.

Catabolism: Process of breaking down muscle tissue.

D

Dietary Fiber: Indigestible plant portion aiding digestion.

Dietary Protein: Protein consumed in the diet.

Dietary Fat: Fat consumed in the diet.

E

Energy: Ability to perform physical work or maintain bodily functions.

Endurance: Sustaining physical activity over time.

Exercise: Physical activity for health and fitness.

F

Fat Loss: Losing body fat.

Fatty Acid: Lipid molecule for energy.

Fiber: Indigestible carbohydrate.

G

Glycogen: Stored carbohydrate in muscles and liver.

Glycogen Depletion: Emptying glycogen stores.

H

HMB (Beta-Hydroxy beta-Methylbutyrate): Anti-catabolic leucine metabolite.

Hormone: Chemical regulating body functions.

Hydration: Consuming fluids for bodily functions.

I

Insulin: Regulates blood sugar levels.

Insulin Resistance: Reduced cell response to insulin.

K

Ketosis: Fat-burning metabolic state.

L

Lactate: Anaerobic exercise byproduct.

Lactate Threshold: Level where lactate accumulates.

M

Macronutrient: Nutrient providing energy.

Meal Frequency: Number of meals per day.

Meal Timing: Timing meals around activities.

N

Nutrient: Necessary substance for body function.

Nutrient Deficiency: Lacking a specific nutrient.

O

Oxidation: Fat breakdown for energy.

P

Phosphocreatine: Muscle energy storage.

R

Resistance Training: Strength-building exercise.

S

Satiety: Feeling full after eating.

Satiety Hormones: Hormones regulating fullness.

T

Thermogenesis: Heat generation, boosting metabolism.

U

Under Recovery: Insufficient rest after exercise.

V

Vitamin: Essential nutrient.

W

Water Loss: Fluid reduction from the body.


Z


Zinc: Important mineral for health.

# REFERENCES

MindBodyGreen. (n.d.). Carb Cycling 101: The Benefits, Drawbacks & Who Should Avoid It. Retrieved from https://www.mindbodygreen.com/articles/carb-cycling-101

Visbody. (n.d.). Carb Cycling 101: The Ultimate Guide to Optimizing Your Fitness. Retrieved from https://visbody.com/blog/carb-cycling-101-the-ultimate-guide-to-optimizing-your-fitness/

Athletic Insight. (n.d.). Carb Cycling: A Beginner's Guide and Meal Plan. Retrieved from https://www.athleticinsight.com/diet/carb-cycling

Noom. (n.d.). What is carb cycling? A beginner's guide (and meal plan). Retrieved from https://www.noom.com/blog/carb-cycling-meal-plan/

Levels Health. (n.d.). What is carb cycling and how does it impact metabolic health? Retrieved from https://www.levelshealth.com/blog/what-is-carb-cycling-and-how-does-it-impact-metabolic-health

Form Nutrition. (n.d.). An Introductory Guide to Carb Cycling and How to Tailor the Method to Your Goals. Retrieved from https://formnutrition.com/inform/an-introductory-guide-to-carb-cycling-and-how-to-tailor-the-method-to-your-goals/

# BONUS WEEKLY PLANNER

Scan the QR code below to get your bonus. Thank you so much for your support. Please, feel free to also support me by dropping a good review for this book on Amazon.